Detoxification: A Clinical Doctor/Patient Manual

by Dr. Richard Schulze

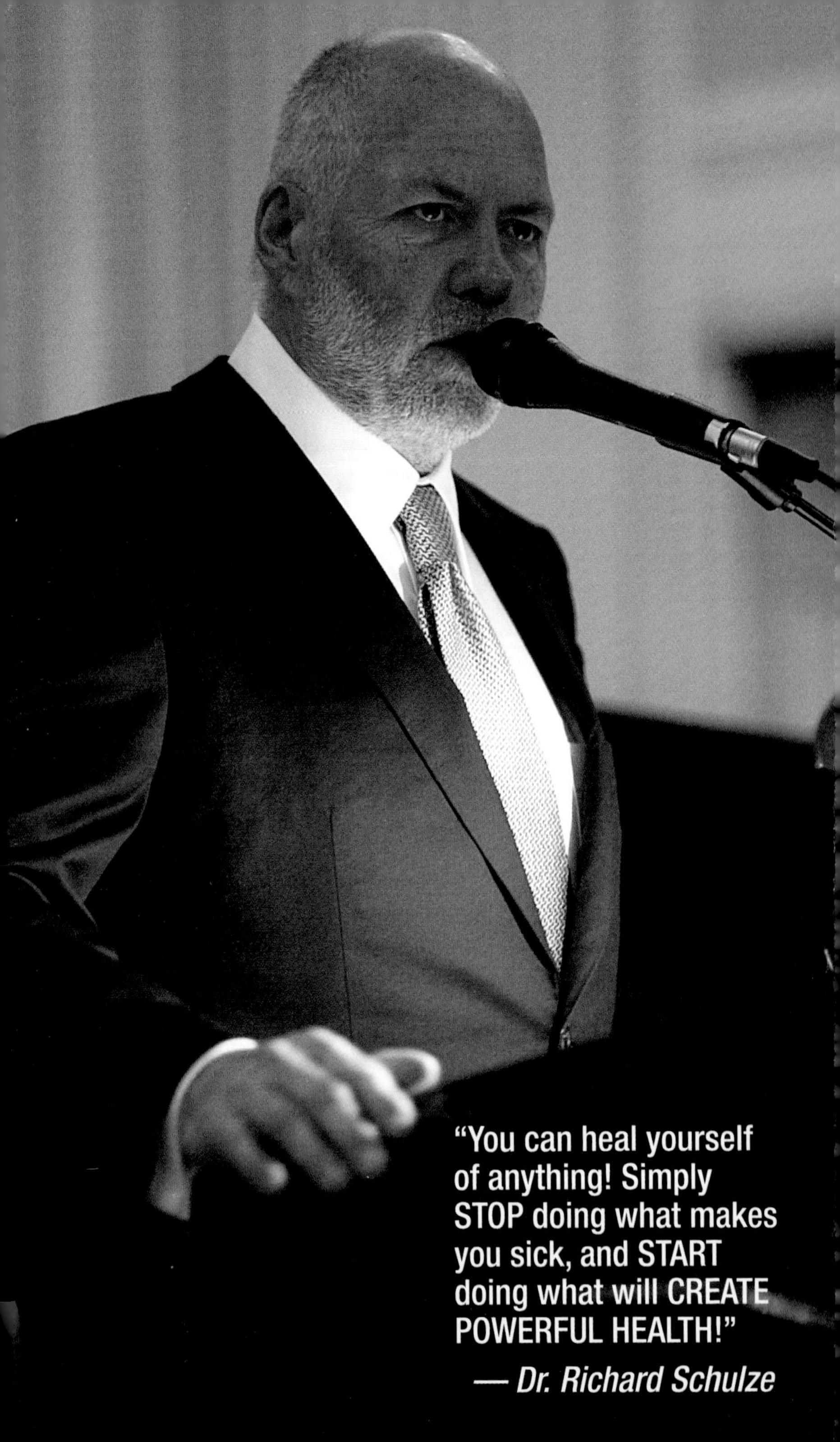
"You can heal yourself of anything! Simply STOP doing what makes you sick, and START doing what will CREATE POWERFUL HEALTH!"
— Dr. Richard Schulze

TABLE OF CONTENTS

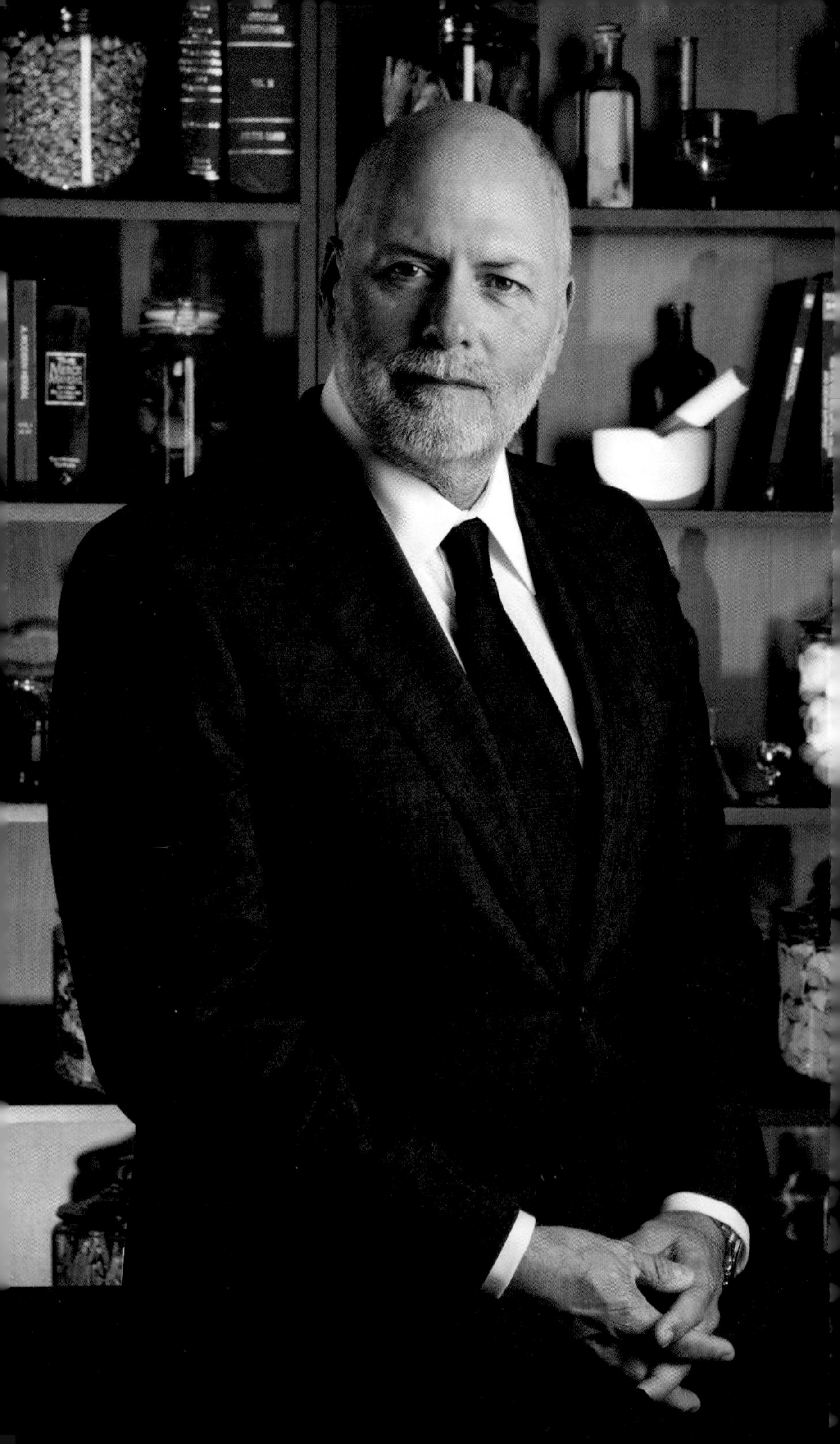

INTRODUCTION

AN INTRODUCTION TO DETOXIFICATION

Most of you know that at the age of 16, the medical doctors told me that I had only a few years to live. They said that by 20, I would be dead, unless I underwent open-heart surgery.

(If you want more details about my healing adventure, go to my BLOG site, www.herbdocblog.com or my website, www.herbdoc.com and read my Biography.)

Mainly, I am happy to announce that I was able to survive, even thrive, and that I am still alive well over 40 years later! But this didn't happen because their diagnosis was incorrect. In fact, it was very correct! It was just that their *prognosis* was wrong.

See, they didn't consider one very important thing, one very important part of the equation… **ME!** I had my powerful spirit, my willingness and my determination to literally do ANYTHING and EVERYTHING in order to help my body heal itself.

So, when I heard *their* answer to my life-threatening problem, which was to crack my chest open, stab a knife into my heart and fill my body with toxic chemicals for the rest of my life, well, I believe that God, the angels or someone or something set off a powerful alarm in my spirit and spoke to me right in that very moment. They told me, "Get the hell out of here or you will be DEAD!" The voice said there was another way, a better way, for me.

In order to avoid a teenage death, and also to avoid open-heart surgery and a lifetime of chemical drugs, I set out on a journey, an adventure, to discover ways, *natural ways*, to stimulate my own body to *heal itself* and to be able to create my own healing miracles. My disease led me on a journey to search out and investigate Healthy and Natural Food Programs, Powerful Elimination Programs, Movement and Exercise Programs, Life-Changing Emotional Programs, and I needed them ALL, and I did them ALL! After all, if I was going to survive, I needed a complete body, mind and spirit makeover!

In my three-year quest to heal myself and heal my heart, without doctors, drugs and hospitals, I also learned a lot about Detoxification.

In my over 40 years of personal experience since then, I have personally done well over 100 intensive Detoxification and Cleansing Programs, from deep Bowel, Liver, Kidney, Lung and Skin Cleansing, to numerous fasts and flushes, some 30-day fasts, and one 60-day fast.

After I healed myself, I traveled worldwide to instruct students in my Detoxification Programs and personally led numerous 3-day, 5-day and also 30-day courses in Cleansing and Detoxification to thousands of people. Even further, I have also guided and assisted tens of thousands of my patients, in my clinic, to do their own detoxification programs, and I learned even more about detoxification when I took my programs to the masses.

The following is a summary of what I learned, what I know, what works, what doesn't and why.

My sole desire is that my work will help you, a family member or a friend, to discover how you can use detoxification programs to do everything from heal the common cold to heal cancer.

— Dr. Schulze

"In the last 40 years, I have personally done well over 100 intensive detoxification and cleansing programs, and I have guided tens of thousands of patients to do theirs!"

"A Detox Program is the antidote for modern living."

CHAPTER 1

WHAT EXACTLY IS A DETOX?

This definition is from the modern, "Dr. Schulze's Dictionary":

"A Detox or Detoxification Program, sometimes also called a Cleanse or a Cleansing program, **is the process of extracting, neutralizing and then eliminating built-up waste, dirt, mucous, sludge, pus, fluids, toxic chemicals, poisons or any harmful residues from your body.** This waste can be in your fat, muscles, organs, cells and even in the various spaces between organs within in your body."

This toxic waste contamination originates from two sources. One source is simply the waste that is generated from the normal and natural metabolic functions of your body, as I will explain in detail later. The second, is from the direct ingestion of toxic chemicals from the food and water that you consume and the air that you breathe, and also from exposure and contamination to toxic environmental chemicals and poisons in our homes, offices, cars and simply by living in the world around us.

Regardless of where these toxins originate, everyone on this planet now has unwanted, potentially harmful and disease-causing waste in their body. And, if this waste is allowed to build up and remain there, it can—and it will—cause irritation, inflammation, scarring, illness, disease and even death.

A Detox Program is the antidote for modern living, especially in modern society. A Detox Program is the ultimate program for Prevention, Preventative Healing and even the Treating

and Healing of Disease. A Detox Program is designed to **draw out** and extract, and even **neutralize,** the accumulated toxic waste and poisons that are in your body. A Detox not only extracts this harmful waste from inside your body, but it also assists your body in the **removal, flushing out** and **elimination** of this waste.

Most often, Detox Programs are targeted to stimulate, flush and clean out your body's own elimination organs. Modern living causes these systems to be susceptible to congestion, constipation, blockage and eventually disease. These systems include your digestive and elimination tract, specifically your colon or large intestine, your liver and gallbladder, and also your urinary tract, your kidneys and your bladder. Detoxification Programs are also used for the cleansing and purification of your blood and lymphatic fluids, and almost every organ and system of your body.

The bottom line is that, just by living life, we naturally manufacture internal waste and additionally we are exposed to and assimilate harmful toxic chemicals in our environment. One of the greatest ways to prevent and even heal disease is to keep ahead of the game by periodically assisting our body in eliminating this built-up toxic waste.

That's a Detox!

"One of the greatest ways to prevent and even heal disease is to keep ahead of the game by periodically assisting our body in eliminating this built-up toxic waste.!"

"There have been over 100,000 new chemicals developed since World War II and less than 2% of them have been studied for safety."

CHAPTER 2

SPECIFICALLY, WHERE DO THESE TOXINS COME FROM?

Source #1: Just Living Creates Metabolic Waste

Every organ and every cell in your body, from your heart and lungs to your brain and nervous system, needs fuel to function and operate. Fuel like vitamins, minerals, amino acids, enzymes, carbohydrates, protein, sugar and fat. And as every organ and *every cell in your body* consumes this fuel, and then functions and does its job—it produces some type of metabolic waste material. Think of it as your body's natural by-product from simply being alive.

Normally, this waste material is eliminated from your body on a regular basis as fecal matter from your bowel, urine from your kidneys, bile and liquid toxins from your liver, sweat from your skin, carbon dioxide from your lungs and on a cellular level, waste from your blood that is picked up and removed by your lymphatic system. **Your body must constantly and continuously eliminate solid, liquid and gaseous waste.**

As you live your life, working, playing, thinking, moving, even resting, your body burns the fuel that you consume and then creates waste that must be eliminated.

Source #2: We Assimilate and Absorb Toxins & Poisons From Our Environment

We assimilate toxic chemicals from our direct exposure to them, from consuming food, drinking water and breathing air.

Food

According to the Food and Drug Administration, the average American grocery cart has well over 100 different highly toxic chemicals in it.

Fast Food, Junk Food, Microwavable Food, Canned Food, Frozen Food, Flash Frozen Food, Dehydrated Food, Reconstituted Food, Convenience Food... this food was once only thought about for disaster survival or space travel, and now it has become the mainstay of the American diet. Fresh food has almost disappeared.

Because almost all modern food is not fresh, it is therefore laden with flavor enhancers, chemical preservatives and artificial colors, sweeteners and additives... the list of added chemicals is almost endless. Pick up almost any food in the grocery store and the list of chemicals and garbage ingredients is usually ten times longer that the main ingredient. Remember when peanut butter was just, well, peanuts? And this doesn't even include the thousands and thousands of chemicals used in the farming, production, preservation and packaging of this food.

Just in the last 100 years, we have consumed and assimilated disease-causing and even lethal amounts of tens of thousands of toxic chemicals while simultaneously watching the disease rates of everything from cancer to neurological diseases skyrocket.

Air

A recent EPA study concluded that air inside American homes is up to **70 TIMES** more polluted than outdoor air, and that toxic fumes from common household cleaners cause cancer.

Here is a short list of TOXINS in the air you are breathing right now... carbon monoxide, lead, ash, soot, ozone, hydrocarbons, nitrogen dioxide, sulfur oxides, insecticides, herbicides and dust from fertilizers and pesticides.

In fact, the air we breathe has less oxygen content today than ever before in history, while it also has the highest concentration of pollution and chemical emissions.

Water

In the average ten-minute shower, the human body absorbs the same amount of CHLORINE as if you drank **20 GALLONS** of tap water.

It has also been declared that there is no water to be found ANYWHERE on the planet anymore that doesn't contain industrial wastes and highly toxic, carcinogenic, mutagenic and disease-causing chemicals, from industrial transformer PCBs to the residues from 10,000 different pharmaceutical drugs.

And Beyond Our Consumption…

There have been over 100,000 new chemicals developed since World War II and less than 2% of them have been studied for safety. Our environment is saturated with poisons from farming chemicals like pesticides and insecticides to industrial chemicals and manufacturing chemicals that are used in making everything from our homes, to what's inside our homes like rugs and furniture, to the clothes we wear, to cleaning chemicals, to the carcinogenic fire retardants in our computers, cell phones and toys. That "new car smell" has now been determined to be the offgassing of over 1,000 toxic chemicals that we use to manufacture the car. We are literally surrounded by poison!

Friends, even in my own business, did you know that almost all organically-grown herbs, after harvesting, are gassed with a highly toxic antibacterial disinfectant called ethylene oxide (ETO), which is a known toxic chemical ***carcinogen*** *and* ***mutagen****? This is a dirty little secret that the herbal manufacturers don't want you to know. And, the herbs can still be labeled Organic and Organically Grown, because they are gassed AFTER they are grown and harvested. By the way, I NEVER EVER use these herbs—actually, I am one of the few manufacturers in the US and the world that refuses to use any chemically-treated herbs, even chemically treated organic herbs, in the production of my herbal medicine. But, my point is even when we do the right thing and make the right choices, we may be still getting poisoned by consuming organic, just usually less poisoned!*

Drug Residues

Drug Residues accumulate in our bodies from the drugs we have taken. The residual remainders of drugs, even the ones we have taken years ago, can still remain in the tissues and cells of our body for years, even decades. And as I mentioned above, our water has residues of 10,000 prescription drugs that other people have taken and either flushed down the toilet or dumped into landfills.

Heavy Metals

Heavy Metals can be from many sources. Many people have mercury contamination from seafood consumption to old tooth fillings, and everything from childhood immunizations to flu shots that are preserved with mercury. We have all been exposed to lead from everything from lead paints to Christmas tree tinsel and to the many toxic, carcinogenic and lethal radioactive materials from X-rays, and now worse, CT scans and MRIs not to mention microwave ovens. The average CT Scan has the same radiation exposure of 442 chest X-rays and leads to over **15,000 deaths EVERY YEAR** from cancer in the USA alone, and causes over 30,000 new cases of cancer annually, making CT Scans one of the highest causes of cancer in America today.

The Bottom Line

Exposure and contamination to toxic and poisonous chemicals is simply a fact of life, especially modern American life. It is the downside of living the American Dream or the negative side to modern living. So in the future, we all need to be a lot more conscious of what we consume, both into our bodies and what we buy and surround ourselves with. And Organic and Recycling are not just hip fads, but they will provide us with a solution to the continual contamination and poisoning of our planet, and protect our children's children's future.

Look, I am NOT trying to depress you, cause an anxiety or panic attack or make you overly paranoid. I believe there is hope and we can and will turn this around, but... at the same time, let's not pretend that everything is OK and that we are not poisoning ourselves with toxic chemicals on a daily basis by eating, drinking, breathing *and living* on this planet.

"Most of my patients didn't even know that their colon wasn't working well, and that they were retaining pounds of fecal sludge, until they did one of my bowel detox programs."

CHAPTER 3

WHY SHOULD YOU CONSIDER DOING A DETOX?

After what I just said, you would be crazy *not* to do a Detox. But some skeptics say we should not need to do detoxification and that our body has built in elimination systems and self-cleansing mechanisms, like self-cleaning ovens. Well, my answer to this is yes it does, this is correct, and under *"normal conditions"* we should NOT need to do any flushing, cleansing or detoxification. But—and here is the big BUT—modern life in America is far from *"normal conditions"*.

So read on, and in this chapter, I will share with you exactly how far we have strayed from normal. And, answering the question as to why you may consider doing a Detox program will reflect back upon the two main categories in the previous Chapter Two: "Where Do These Toxins Come From?"—internal build-up of metabolic waste and environmental toxic exposure.

68,952 Bowel Movements Short

In Chapter Two, under Source #1: Metabolic Waste, I stated that "normally" this waste material is eliminated from your body on a regular basis. I repeat:

"Normally, this waste material is eliminated from your body on a regular basis as fecal matter from your bowel, urine from your kidneys, bile and liquid toxins from your liver, sweat from your skin, carbon dioxide from your lungs and on a cellular level, waste from your blood that is picked up and removed by your lymphatic system. ***Your body must constantly and continuously eliminate solid, liquid and gaseous waste.****"*

The key word here is **"normally"**.

Let's start with the main solid-waste removal system in our bodies, the colon. In America, every book (from modern high school health books to medical texts) states that it is "normal" to have one bowel movement three to five times a week.

But, in my extensive worldwide travels visiting primitive people—who live in very remote areas, eat simple natural foods (mostly raw food, high fiber and low fat/cholesterol diets), get plenty of exercise and have very low amounts of stress—well, I have noticed that these people have one bowel movement a day, for every major meal that they eat. And, most of them ate three main meals a day. So, most of them were "popping a squat" (my native term for having a bowel movement) three times a DAY, not three to five times a week. *The difference in this frequency adds up to a startling number...*

While we are having three to five bowel movements a week (let's say an average of four a week) times 52 weeks in a year (208 total), times the average lifespan of 78 years, we are having about 16,224 bowel movements on average during our lifespan.

On the other hand, the primitive natives are having about three bowel movements a day, seven days a week. This equals 21 bowel movements a week, times 52 weeks in a year, which equals 1,092 bowel movements a year, times 78 years, and that equals 85,176 total bowel movements on average during their lifespan.

The difference? We are 68,952 Bowel Movements SHORT!!!

That means we are Sixty-Eight Thousand Nine Hundred and Fifty-Two Bowel Movements SHORT in our lifetime!

Medical doctors and health authorities in America might say this is "normal", but what is also "normal" in America is the highest incidence of colon and rectal cancer in the world.

In just the past 50 years, we have watched the incidence of constipation and colon disease rise dramatically. Most of my patients didn't even know that their colon wasn't working well, and that they were retaining pounds of fecal sludge, until they did one of my bowel detox programs. I had many patients that only went once week, and even once a month. If you are into this kind of Guinness World Record of dysfunctional constipated bowel thing, then I highly suggest that you get my book on my 5-Day Bowel Detox Program and read about my record breaking patients. I am sure you will find it highly amusing. This information will also be included into Volume Two of my Detoxification series.

To reflect this, I will quote the Merck Manual, the esteemed international standard medical text for the diagnosis and prognosis of disease...

Their statistics state that in 1950, 10% of all Americans had diverticulosis, or herniated sacs, in their colon caused by the pressure and stuffing of constipation, where fecal matter literally pushes into a weak part in the wall of the colon, herniates the wall creating a saccular bubble, and stays there. But, in 1955, they raised that to 15%. And in 1972, they went up to 30%, and in the 1987 edition, they said just about half of Americans have diverticulosis or herniated sacs in their colon.

In the most recent edition of the Merck Manual it states, if people live long enough, EVERY American will have herniated bowel pockets or diverticuli. And, basic common sense will tell you it just stays in there. In fact, the whole colon can get encased in fecal matter in advanced constipation, to where it looks like a rusty pipe, an old steel or galvanized pipe in your house, and when you look through it you can only see a small hole.

Note: Some of you may think that primitive people don't have the same longevity as people living in modern civilized society. Well, think again. The United States spends more money per person annually on medical care, and **doesn't even come into the top**

15 countries worldwide for longevity and lifespan. Obviously, we are not getting the most bang for our buck.

Modern Life Causes the MALFUNCTION of Your Waste Elimination Organs

Modern life also disrupts and negatively affects the ability of the Liver and Gallbladder, the Kidneys and Bladder, the Lungs, the Skin and the Lymphatic System from their doing their roles of routinely cleansing your body of toxins, waste, and then efficiently eliminating it.

The Liver

Fatty foods, fried foods and a diet high in cholesterol (because they are based on animal foods) causes your liver and gallbladder to get congested, to the point that the fatty sludge literally coagulates and turns into stones in your gallbladder (gallstones) and even liver. Alcohol and drug use, even prescription and over the counter drugs like Acetaminophen, are all known to cause fatty livers, cirrhosis and even liver cell rupture and bleeding, and eventually hepatocellular necrosis (liver cell death). Every chemical that we come in contact with, whether from our food or from our environment, ALL must be broken down, processed, neutralized and eliminated by your liver. The contamination of modern life and modern living has overworked and overloaded our livers to the point where they no longer can do their basic job of filtering our blood of chemicals to protect us. This has led many medical researchers, oncologists and scientists to believe that modern life's chemical bombardment of the liver, and the liver's inability to keep up with this toxic bombardment, thus allowing toxic chemicals to remain in our blood and body, is the major factor leading to the increased incidence of almost every disease, especially cancer.

The Kidneys

The high consumption of soft drinks, alcohol, coffee, black tea, and also drugs and chemicals, has also taken a drastic toll on our urinary system. This hinders, congests, slows down and scars the kidneys and bladder and impairs them from doing their job of removing the acids, impurities and liquid waste from our blood and body. The incidence of patients needing kidney dialysis and kidney transplants has skyrocketed over the past decade, and the sales of adult diapers have become a $250 million dollar industry.

The Lungs

Smoking, second-hand smoke, industrial air pollution and chemical off-gassing have all had a very negative impact on our lungs. Not only do they clog the tiny cells in our lungs that enable us to assimilate precious oxygen, but also inhibit our ability to eliminate waste gasses like carbon dioxide.

The Skin

Many don't think of our skin as an elimination organ, but actually it is the largest elimination organ in our body. Your skin (if it is clean and healthy) can eliminate up to 10 pounds of liquids, gasses and even solids in one day. For many reasons, from the harsh soaps and detergents we use, to the clothes we wear, to the lotions and potions we apply to our skin, our skin gets clogged and suffocated, and therefore cannot do its job as an elimination organ. This too contributes to the back up and retention of toxins and poisons in our body.

Modern Living Causes the OVERLOADING of Your Waste Elimination Organs

Modern living is a toxic chemical bombardment. You are exposed to more toxins, they are more concentrated toxins, and you now get more frequent exposure.

With modern living, we are simply exposed to more toxic chemicals than ever before in history, and worse, at a much higher concentration and at a faster rate than our body can process, neutralize or eliminate them. As I stated earlier, this is primarily due to a food program that has more toxins, more poisons and less fiber in it, than ever before in history. We have junk food on almost every major street corner. Candy, cookies and chips are our snack food. French fries (another name for rancid trans fat grease sticks) are the most eaten vegetable in America. Even if you don't eat out and only shop at grocery stores, you are still filling yourself with insecticides, preservatives, colorings, flavor enhancers... the list of chemical additives is almost endless. Even if you buy only Organic, Vegan, *health food*, the processing and packaging is still often toxic.

Secondly, modern living means that we are moving our bodies less now than ever before in history. Due to everything from modern transportation to computers, we are sitting on our asses more and not moving much for the most of the day. Exercise alone stimulates the digestive and elimination systems, including the bowel and the liver, promoting the elimination of waste. It creates better circulation, because it moves bodily fluids like blood and lymphatic fluid, and causes better elimination of carbon dioxide from the lungs and flushes sweat from the skin. Moving our body helps to eliminate more waste and toxins from our body and helps to do it more efficiently and effectively. But we are moving less, not more.

Also, in Chapter Two, I talked about the onslaught from chemical pollution, from simply living in America today. Everything from the over 100,000 new industrial chemicals that have been invented since World War II, to your "new car smell" being the off-gassing of over 1,000 different toxic chemicals. I think you get the picture. Modern life and modern living in America today exposes us to unprecedented levels of toxic chemicals.

Well then, it doesn't take a genius to see that our bodies are now being bombarded and polluted with more toxins than ever before in history. And consequently, our body's natural elimination organs are overworked and overloaded, having to process this toxic chemical onslaught.

The Bottom Line

For ALL of the reasons I have previously mentioned, and many, many more, modern life and modern living has overloaded, overworked, polluted, hindered, irritated, inflamed, clogged, scarred, constipated, degenerated, maimed and diseased all of your bodies major elimination organs and systems.

This has caused a slowing down effect of your body's natural elimination of toxic waste, and caused this waste to be backed up, being deposited and even stored in your muscles, fat, organs, cells and the inner spaces of your body.

This backup, storage and retention of waste in our bodies pollutes us. It overworks and eventually depresses our immune system, which lowers our resistance to disease. It poisons us, it kills cells, it weakens any organ where it is deposited and therefore can cause ANY illness or disease.

For all of these reasons, this unavoidable toxic consequence of modern life and modern living underscores the serious importance of regular and routine Cleansing and Detoxification, and also the importance of toning and protecting these precious elimination organs and systems.

"DETOXIFICATION Heals Illness and Disease And Creates Powerful Health!"

"Natural Healing is as old as the people on this planet. It is the original form of healing, the same as herbs are the original medicine on this planet, from the beginning of time."

CHAPTER 4

THE BEGINNING: MY PERSONAL DETOX ADVENTURES

Shortly after I received my "death sentence" from my team of cardiologists, I felt screwed. Here I was a teenager, my parents were both dead, and now I was being told I was going to die very soon. So, I either had to give up and just die, or suck it up and get to work. I decided to suck it up. Feeling sorry for myself didn't feel like a positive or healing option, and I was scared to death. So again, sucking it up and getting to work sounded like the best option to me.

I remember in school (in science class) I was taught that the human body was a self-repairing and self-healing machine. But, my medical doctors told me that this would be impossible in my case, and that nothing, NOTHING would keep me alive but surgery.

But, could my body possibly heal itself? Could my body possibly correct what was wrong? I believed that it could, and the alternative was so damn frightening to me, actually horrifying, so again, I decided to get to work.

I decided that in order to stimulate, to promote and to push my body into doing something that the medical doctors said was impossible, to create some kind of natural healing miracle, I needed to make my body the most aggressive, powerful and effective self-healing machine possible—more than any normal person.

So I started reading the most unusual, alternative, way out and extreme books on self-healing and natural healing that I could find, and implementing these various programs into my life.

Look, my alternative was death, so if someone told me to eat donkey shit mixed with carrot juice, I did it, and smiled!

I had already started on a vegetarian food program, which naturally (because of the increased fiber and less fat and cholesterol) got my bowel working much better. Then, I added a few bowel cleansing herbs, and I was going great. Next, I became a vegan. I dramatically increased my movement by getting very involved in the Martial Arts and Yoga, as much as I could handle, constantly pushing myself. I also started investigating many different types of psychotherapy and meditation to cleanse and detoxify my mind.

But, from the alternative healing books I was reading, I also knew that it was time to begin some type of serious detoxification program. With my history of constipation, current low level of health and medical death sentence, I decided that a maximum level of detoxification was necessary.

So, I picked up more books on alternative health and healing, and started out to try some popular Detox routines of the 1960s. There was Arnold Ehret's *Rational Fasting* (he was born 1866), Paul Braggs' *Miracle of Fasting* (he was born in 1895) and the classic work by Herbert Sheldon, *Fasting Can Save Your Life* (he was also born in 1895) and many others. But, they were all Detox *Antiques.*

Natural Healing is as old as the people on this planet. It is the original form of healing, the same as herbs are the original medicine on this planet, from the beginning of time. There are references to it in the Bible and every spiritual book ever written. Even John Wesley (the founder of the Methodist church) wrote a book he called *Primitive Physic* back in 1747. He was a huge promoter of Nature Cure and Natural Healing using everything from fruit fasts to enemas.

Now don't get me wrong, the fundamental principles of "Nature Cure" and "Natural Healing", which have their modern American roots in Traditional European Medicine and were brought to America by the early immigrants and settlers of America, (including John Wesley) are rock solid powerful healing fundamentals.

But, I was looking for more up-to-date information. After all, life in the 1960s in America was rapidly changing and different from the cowboy times of the 1880s or the trench wars of World War I. Junk food restaurants were opening up on every street corner in America, so I figured there may be many *upgrades* to this older healing technology.

The Beginning: My First Detox

I did my first Detox following the advice of Herbert Sheldon; from his book *Fasting Can Save Your Life*. I found his water fast very difficult to do, and after three days I felt so dizzy, sick and intoxicated, I could barely communicate with others or drive a car safely. It was very rough and I felt terrible. I am not saying that it was not effective—I am just saying that I needed to be like Jesus and go off into the woods for 40 days as there was absolutely NO WAY I could do anything but sit in my room, drink water and stare at the walls. And, I had to stop all my other healing programs while doing this fast, so this was not a great way to get well. Additionally, most of the Natural Hygienists that I met promoting this program were antiques themselves, over 70 years old, and I was a young teenage hippie, so I simply felt there must be a better way.

So, I started following other health gurus and alternative doctors' programs, and moved more into juice fasting instead of water fasting, and I had much greater results. It was also very detoxifying and I eliminated a huge amount of toxins and poisons doing various fruit and vegetable juice fasts, including lots of water, and also herbal teas. I was doing intensive deep cleaning, but also the minimal nutrition in the juices allowed me to keep doing Martial Arts and Yoga, and gave me plenty of energy to do all of the rest of my healing programs. I also found that with various juices I could stimulate different elimination organs. I used prune and apple for more effective bowel cleansing, watermelon or lemons and limes for more effective kidney and bladder cleansing, and also the herbs ginger and garlic, mixed with citrus juices and olive oil to flush my liver and gallbladder. Using various juices for flushing not only supplied my body with vitamins, minerals, enzymes, amino acids and live food energy, they also helped to draw out and flush toxins right out of my body.

The bottom line is that after three years on my health program, new lifestyle and many, many detox programs, fasts and flushes, I totally healed my heart and was given a clean bill of health. Again, for more details, check my bio.

So the bottom line, Juice Fasting for me was a powerfully effective detoxification program. Because of the increased nutrition, instead of sitting in my room like a zombie all day, it allowed me to continue my physical activity and gave me all the energy I needed to do all of my other healing programs. In fact, on the 27th day of one of my 30-day juice fasts, I kickboxed 16 rounds of full contact kickboxing, and I was so fast, people commented that they couldn't even see it when I hit them—now that's ENERGY!

The next obvious step to me, seemed to be to learn more about fasting and detoxification, and as I was learning more, people were naturally drawn to me after hearing my story, and asked me if I could help them. So, I helped them heal themselves from their diseases. Basically, I became a doctor by accident. But, I wanted even more.

I searched out and interned with the best Natural Healing doctors of my time, like the very famous Dr. Bernard Jensen, graduating from his school and then interning with him at his famous Hidden Valley Health ranch. I also studied with and eventually apprenticed with the most famous living American clinical master herbalist of this era, Dr. John Ray Christopher. Eventually, he gave me a great honor and asked me to teach with him at his school where I did up until his death in the early 1980s, and continued for a decade after. I also stalked and studied with the icon of European Nature Cure, Paavo Airola, and also closely followed the teachings of the great Dr. Randolph Stone, Dr. Ann Wigmore, Henry Lindlahr, Benedict Lust, Norman Walker, Tilden, Kniepp, Priznitz… and many, many others.

So, I want to state right here, that even though I stopped following some of these doctors specific instructions, and changed, upgraded, bastardized, modernized, cannibalized and even metamorphosed their works, I honor and respect ALL of these great Natural Healers, Nature Cure doctors and teachers, scientists and religious leaders and gurus before me—because without their amazing work, I would not be here today, I WOULD NOT BE ALIVE TODAY! I am the living descendent of all of these great masters and I have simply added my life's personal and clinical *upgrades* and *modernization* to their work.

Many of these great men and women were more than ridiculed. Even in their own time, they were attacked by organized religious groups, medical associations and even government agencies. Some were imprisoned numerous times, some were even beaten, and a few died in prison. But, ALL of them stayed true to their Natural Healing Crusade until their death.

They ALL were AWESOME, and I am so honored and humbled to be a descendent of these great masters, a link in their work, and continuing their work!

OK, so after training, studying, apprenticing and interning with the more current natural doctors I mentioned above, and doing over 100 various detoxification, fasting, flushing and cleansing routines myself, including 30-day and 60-day juice fasts, and also from leading my tens of thousands of patients in my clinic through numerous detoxification and cleansing routines, well, I think I understand Detoxification and Cleansing, and Juice Flushing and Raw Food Programs, maybe better than anyone I've met.

"Flushing not fasting worked much better with my patients, and in my clinic, as it gave a more accurate description, impression and visual of what I wanted them to achieve."

CHAPTER 5

FLUSHING NOT FASTING

WORDS are very powerful, maybe all-powerful. As Louise Hay says, "Every thought you think, and every WORD you speak, creates your future". So in my clinic, I not only developed new programs that proved to be more powerful and effective healing programs, but I also took it on myself to change some of the *language* of Natural Healing that was hundreds of years old or older.

For instance, I never liked the word "diet". To me, I see only DIEt, and I don't want to die just yet. In fact, I often talk about my *Game*, "Quality and Quantity". I would get my patients to play this game with me, which is to live our lives in such a way that we feel great and have tons of energy to do all of the things we want to do, and to do them for as long as we possibly can. This is the game, and we want to win it by **feeling great, having endless energy and living as long as possible.** So again, I don't want to see the word DIEt, especially when I am eating!

Arnold Ehret, a great Natural Healing pioneer, had a food program he called the *Mucousless Diet Healing Program*, and again, I don't want to think about *removing mucous* while I am eating, *please*. So, over the past 40 years, I have done some *name changing* to better suit my *positive* Natural Healing lifestyle.

I also never liked the word fasting, from doing my first fast. It felt to me like deprivation or starvation and I like to eat—wait a minute, I LOVE to eat! And wait another minute, on every water or juice fast I did, the liquid wasn't restricted. In fact, most healers suggested to almost drown yourself, that the water and the juices were dissolving the toxins and flushing them away. The more you drink, the more you flush. Wait a minute—flush, flushing, FLUSHING! This is more like it.

First, it better describes what I want you to do, and secondly, it sounds lavish to me, like I get to have all that I want, not like deprivation, more like abundance!

So from that point on, I dropped using the word "fasting" and started using the word FLUSHING.

It also worked much, much better in the clinic with my patients, as it gave a more accurate description, impession and visual of what I wanted them to achieve.

So, when we get to the chapter on my Three Clinical Food Programs, you will see that my most detoxifying food program is simply called "Juice *Flushing*".

"I have found that 5-Day Detox Programs, done Monday through Friday are for the most part, the best timing to ensure a successful Detox."

CHAPTER 6
WHEN IS THE BEST TIME TO DO A DETOX?

It has now been over 40 years since the medical doctors told this teenage child that he would soon die. For those of you that have been at death's door and *survived,* I know that you will understand when I say I now realize that this "death sentence" was my "greatest gift". I am beyond eternally thankful for this experience.

Unknown to me in the beginning, when I had to stop my self-pity, suck it up and get to work, well, I had no idea then that my inherited heart disease would eventually take me on the greatest of all adventures, not only into my own healing, but way, way beyond that. This 40-year life adventure that my "heart" took me on includes operating my own Natural Healing and Herbal Medicine Clinic that spanned three decades, helping tens of thousands of patients to heal themselves *naturally*. This adventure took me for a 20-year ride, teaching Natural Healing and Herbal Medicine at colleges and retreats worldwide, and also helping my graduate students establish their own clinics. This adventure—my own healing and my patients' healings—taught me what works and what doesn't, and it was the event that led me to develop all of my Clinical Herbal Medicines and Natural Healing Programs and Routines.

So, why am I saying all of this now? Because I want you to know that I have learned a few things. And, as I have said before, I have learned what WORKS and what doesn't, especially when it comes to doing a Detox. And this leads me into…

When is the best time to do a Detox? OK, for this discussion, I need to divide all of you up into two groups, based on WHY you are doing a Detox: Prevention or Healing?

Group One: Detoxification for PREVENTION

These are people that are well and that are doing a Detox Program for preventative health reasons. They are not sick, they feel fine, and they want to remain that way.

For this group, I can tell you what I did with all of my patients…

In my clinic, for my patients that were healthy, I instructed them to do Seasonal Detoxification Programs for about a week in length, four times a year, to periodically flush out and prevent the build-up of waste and toxins in their body, while stimulating and toning their body's elimination organs and keeping them in healthy working order.

So, I suggest for anyone in this category, to do a 5-Day Detoxification Program, once every season, four times a year.

I always start with the colon (a Bowel Detoxification) and I explain why I suggest this in detail in Step 3 of Chapter Eight. And, I suggest doing this in the **Spring**, to do some effective "spring cleaning" and to get all the old waste out from your winter hibernation and stagnation.

In the Summer, I usually suggest either a Liver/Gallbladder Detox, or a Kidney/Bladder Detox. This can depend on anything from whether the person has a family history of liver *or* kidney ailments, to whether they have brown eyes (do the Liver) or blue eyes (do the Kidney), or just whatever they feel in the mood for.

In the Fall, I would suggest the second Bowel Detox of the year, to get your major elimination organ clean before the coming winter.

And in the Winter, I suggest starting whichever Detox (the Liver or the Kidney) that they did not do in the summer.

Group Two: Detoxification for HEALING Disease and Illness

If a person is not feeling well, or has any illness or disease, then the best time to start their Detoxification is IMMEDIATELY! RIGHT NOW!

This is also the time that the person should stop eating all foods and start flushing, as suggested in Chapter Nine on my 3 Clinical Food Programs.

YOU have to be the person to judge the type of Detox, the length of the Detox and the intensity of the Detox, which should be based on the severity of your illness or disease.

If you have digestive or elimination problems, like gas, bloating, gastric reflux, indigestion, heartburn, nausea, colic, vomiting all the way to constipation, irritable bowel syndrome, Crohn's disease, spastic colon or something similar to this, then start with a 5-Day Detox for the Bowel. Or, do a 5-Day Detox for the Liver and Gallbladder if your complaints are more digestive and not bowel-related. I would even suggest to do one followed by the other, in either order. That's right, do a 5-Day Detox for the Bowel the first week and then a 5-Day Detox for the Liver and Gallbladder the following week. You can even double-up and do two 5-Day Detox Programs for the Bowel or Liver. There are no hard and fast rules here, except that you keep doing your Detox Program until you feel better, until the pain is gone, until you are not aware you have the problem anymore or until the problem is GONE!

The same would go for a urinary tract infection of the kidneys or bladder. You would choose the 5-Day Detox for the Kidneys and Bladder and, if necessary, do a second Detox the following week, and even a third or fourth Detox, if the problem persists.

For any serious disease such as Diabetes, or even Heart Disease or Cancer, the minimum I suggest is a 30-Day Detoxification Program. These are chronic and life-threatening diseases that took years to manifest themselves and become clinically detectable in your body. You not only need to do a serious 30-Day Detoxification, you should consider doing my *new* Incurables Program, which is a 90-Day Detox. The name for this program implies any disease that allopathic medicine considers "incurable", which are most diseases from Arthritis and Alzheimer's to Diabetes, Heart Disease, Cancer and so on. All of these Detox Programs are described in the next book, *Detoxification: Volume Two.*

Why FIVE Days?

Early in my own personal Detox experience, I used to think that a good time to do a Detox Program would be the weekends, as did most of my patients, when we are off work. But, more often than not, right in the middle of my Saturday morning juicing, a friend would call me and invite me to a party that night, where all of my friends were going to be, and I would show up with my lemon water. Two bad things would almost always happen. One, my friends would think I was a pompous health fanatic, like I was doing this to show off or to get attention, or to make myself look better than them. No one in the midst of a party, eating party food and drinking sodas or alcohol, wants to be reminded that the food and drink they are consuming is toxic. This is not a way to build friendships. And, even if no one said anything to me, I noticed after a year, my party invitations were few and far between.

Secondly, and worse, often I couldn't resist the sugar and would go from three days on lemon water to using my lemon water to wash down three pieces of chocolate birthday cake and send my body into a toxic sugar shock and a digestive nightmare and feel horrible for the next few days. Either way, weekend Detox programs usually don't give you the results you are looking for, physically, mentally or *socially.*

So, I soon discovered that the best time to do a Detox Program was actually *during* the week, while at work. Keeping myself busy at work made time fly by and it was easy to prepare my juices, teas, herbs and anything else I needed and take it in a sports bottle or a

Stanley stainless steel thermos, and throw it all into my backpack. I was much more successful at completing 5-Day Detox Programs during the week at work, then attempting to do any type of weekend Detox.

In the clinic, this experience mirrored my patients' experiences. Most of my patients were in the movie, television or entertainment community. They worked hard and usually long hours. Doing their Detox Programs during the week made them fly by, almost effortlessly.

Also, for the average person, five days is about the right amount of time to do some great cleaning and detoxification.

So the bottom line is that I have found that 5-Day Detox Programs, done Monday through Friday are for the most part, the best timing to ensure a successful Detox. Also, for the average person, it is enough time to unplug that gallbladder, flush out the bowel or even heal that nasty kidney or bladder infection. And if it isn't, just do another 5-Day Detox the very next week.

Now having said that, I am talking mainly about doing a 5-Day Detox for general seasonal cleansing and the prevention of disease—NOT necessarily treating disease. When treating disease, generally you stop all work, stay home and begin your Detox immediately (regardless of the day of the week) and probably rest for a day or two and follow it up with an additional 5-Day Detox, just to make absolutely sure you have effectively dealt with the issue and completely healed yourself.

Which takes me right to the next chapter, **"Chapter Seven: What Will Happen When You Do A Detox?"**

"There is nothing more empowering than healing yourself, without doctors, drugs and hospitals, but instead, doing it YOURSELF!"

CHAPTER 7

WHAT WILL HAPPEN WHEN YOU DO A DETOX?

What YOU will notice by doing a Detox...

Doing a Detox not only removes backed-up, accumulated and stored waste, toxins and poisons from your body, but it also keeps you healthier and cleaner by making your body a more efficient elimination machine.

When your body gets clean and your elimination systems are cleaned, flushed, toned, strengthened and *tuned-up*, three things happen...

#1: Problems Go Away

I would love to tell you that I always knew what was wrong with my patients when they came to my clinic, but the truth is most of the time I didn't have a clue. According to the medical industry's own studies, the top medical clinics in the world, with their trillions of dollars worth of high-tech machinery, are still less than 25% correct with their disease diagnosis. So, little old me in my simple little clinic at the beach didn't have a chance.

This is why I love Natural Healing so much, because it doesn't really matter if I knew what was wrong with my patients, let alone knew how to fix them. I knew that **their own body would heal itself,** from whatever was wrong with them, from whatever disease they had—their body would know what was wrong and how to heal itself.

It is so simple, yet so foolproof. In the first week in medical school, you learn that one of the most basic, yet primary functions of the human body is to repair and heal *itself.* **I knew my patients' bodies wanted to be well, they just weren't up to this self-healing task, because they were run down, not getting enough help, and to top it all off, they were dirty machines.**

I knew that all I had to do was get them to STOP killing themselves, get healthier, and clean up this dirty mess inside that was the result of years (probably decades) of unhealthy living.

I had to simply assist their body to get into a cleaner, healthier and stronger state, where their body turns its own self-healing mechanisms back on. **Simply put, your body wants to naturally heal itself; it just needs the opportunity to do so! It needs your help.**

The best way to assist your body to want to heal itself is simply to get healthy, by creating a healthy lifestyle… **because Creating Powerful Health Naturally Eliminates Disease.** The Chinese have an old saying, *"Focus on the GOOD to Eliminate the BAD"*, and that is exactly what Natural Healing is. Hanging in my clinic, and now in my herbal pharmacy, is a sign that reads, **"You can heal yourself of ANYTHING, ANY DISEASE. Just STOP doing what created your illness, and START doing what will Create Powerful Health!"** It doesn't get any simpler than that!

So, I would get my patients to do all of my Detox Programs, and then also Eat Right, Breathe Deeper, Move More, and teach and train them to develop a Positive Attitude, and sure enough, their body would begin to heal itself.

There isn't any disease or condition of the human body that isn't helped by getting healthier *and getting cleaner.* In my clinic, I personally witnessed every ailment and disease known to mankind reverse and heal itself by cleansing the body and creating a healthy lifestyle.

Detoxification is one of the first steps in any healing program and process, that gets all of the accumulated and stored waste and

toxins out of the body, tones up all of our elimination organs and systems, and triggers your natural self-healing response.

#2: Again, Problems Go Away

Rarely does anyone choose to go to a "weed doctor" first. Almost all of my patients had been to many doctors, clinics, emergency rooms and medical specialists, before they ever called my office for an appointment. Many had also visited the most prestigious medical clinics in the world like the Mayo Clinic and Stanford University Medical Center. In fact, most of them had also exhausted all of the local *alternative* doctors such as chiropractors, naturopaths, homeopaths, acupuncturists and oriental and Ayurvedic medical doctors, even other herbalists and religious, faith and energy healers. Many had even tried psychiatry and psychotherapy, because eventually when you cannot be well some doctor somewhere will suggest that "it is all in your head". But, they were all still sick when they walked into my clinic door!

Anyway, again what made my approach unique is that I never tried to heal my patients or their dis-eases. Instead, I put them on all of my Detox Programs to flush the waste out of their bodies, and then helped them to create a very healthy life and lifestyle, physically, emotionally and even spiritually, and when the power of these Detox Programs and this new healthy lifestyle "kicked in", well, their diseases just simply disappeared.

No matter how far removed a disease may seem, no matter how unrelated or distant it may seem from simple Detoxification, when you get clean and get healthy, your body will find that problem, and get rid of it and repair itself and heal itself, period.

Let me give you a few brief examples...

I remember one woman had supposedly incurable migraine headaches. She had been to every medical doctor and specialist for migraines and even special migraine treatment clinics and experimental university medical programs, and additionally to over 20 alternative doctors trying to cure her migraines. And she still had them! By the way, they ALL just looked at her head!

Well, in the first few minutes of my consultation, I looked at her ass instead. Seriously, I asked a few of my beginning questions and quickly discovered that she was, and had been, severely constipated all of her life. She was barely having one bowel movement a week (if not one every two weeks) and had been this way for years—actually decades. I didn't need to ask any more questions. I started her *immediately* on my 5-Day Detox for the Bowel and in just a few days, her migraines were gone and never came back. Her migraines were caused by internal poisoning from years of built-up waste and toxins in her body.

I had another woman who was actually scheduled to have her back nerves cut, because she had been in severe back pain, constantly for three years, and no drug, no medical doctor, and even no chiropractor, physical therapist and even yoga or massage was able to help her. After one 5-Day Bowel Detox she never had back pain again. Think about it? The bowel lies right against the spine.

I had a man whose life had come to a total standstill with chronic depression so bad that on his first visit he was driven to my clinic by his family. He couldn't speak, except he kept shouting "NO!", and he couldn't take his hands away from covering his face. He had been a brilliant professor, but for a year now he had been an emotional cripple, and his team of medical doctors said there was no hope. After ONLY Bowel Detoxification and no other programs, he was completely healed and went back to work—his depression was completely gone!

I have thousands of stories like this and you will find many more of them in Volume Two and in my Bowel, Liver and Kidney Detox programs. I am always AMAZED by not only the power of Detoxification, but also how it can heal so many seemingly unrelated diseases. And, this is simply because when you are filled with toxic poison, this poison can affect, infect and disrupt the function of ANY organ or ANY system in your body and make it sick. Consequently, when you do a thorough Detox program, you can expect ANY healing miracle to happen.

#3: ENERGY, ENERGY, ENERGY, ENERGY, ENERGY!

When toxins, poisons, waste, acids and mucous are flushed and removed from your body and from your organs, tissues and cells, you will feel great. And, one of the most noticeable ways you will feel great is you will have a lot more energy.

Your immune system will be able to rest and recharge, instead of constantly fighting off bacteria and pathogens that are built-up in your body. Your liver will say a big thank you and be able to rest more instead of processing poison 24/7/365. And, a healthy liver gives you more energy.

There are literally hundreds of reasons why, when you clean up your body and get your elimination organs working more efficiently, that you will notice that you have an abundance of energy.

In fact, one of the most common responses and comments I would hear from my patients was that they felt 25 years younger, because they now had more energy than they have ever felt in their lives.

The reason is simple. After a Detox your body is clean, clear and operates more efficiently. It uses its fuel better and more efficiently, it eliminates its waste faster and the blockages have been removed. Your immune system gets stronger, and every internal organ benefits. All of this contributes to feeling great and having an abundance of energy.

My patients all also told me they felt powerful *and that they were empowered.* There is nothing more empowering than healing yourself, without doctors, drugs and hospitals, but instead, doing it YOURSELF!

"Bowel Detoxification is the FIRST and most important step in any healing program and the FIRST Detoxification that EVERYONE needs to do."

CHAPTER 8
THE FIRST THREE STEPS IN HEALING ANY ILLNESS OR DISEASE

And Creating Powerful Health

In my own healing adventure and again in the clinic, I was constantly reminded of a few things. You could call these three basic fundamentals of Natural Healing, but to me they are much more, they are gems, they are pearls of wisdom.

Step 1: STOP EATING

The first one is, if you are sick, STOP EATING and go straight to Juice Flushing. You will be reminded of this again in the very next chapter, "Chapter Nine: My 3 Clinical Food Programs", what they are, and even more important, when to use them.

Is it starve a cold and feed a fever? Or, starve a fever and feed a cold? IT'S STARVE EVERYTHING!

Is it which foods and food programs are better for which ailments, illnesses or diseases? Is it macrobiotic, fish/chicken, vegetarian, vegan, fruitarian or McDonalds? NONE of them! If you are ill, **STOP EATING** and go immediately onto Pure Water, Herbal Teas and Fresh Organic Raw Fruit and Vegetable Juices and flood yourself with them—FLUSH YOURSELF!

And DO NOT even think of eating ANYTHING until you are at least feeling much better, if not totally healed.

Any animal knows enough to stop eating when they are feeling ill; any animal, except humans.

Step 2: GET POSITIVE

Nothing Positive ever happens when you are being Negative. I will repeat that. **Nothing Positive ever happens when you are being Negative, so *GET POSITIVE RIGHT NOW.***

My patients used to drag themselves into my clinic, carrying boxes of paperwork, to almost prove to me that they in fact did have the specific disease that they said they had. Boxes of blood test results, allergy test results, ultrasounds, X-rays, CT Scans, MRI reports, electro cardiograms, even DVDs of their echo-cardiograms, pathology reports, biopsy reports, letters from their medical doctors, letters from supposed medical specialists and the top clinics in the world, second opinions, third opinions, fourth opinions, letters from their psychics, whatever, all to show me—to prove to me what was wrong with them.

But, now they were dying and all the medical doctors, all of the specialists and all of the tests, couldn't save them now. All the treatments had failed and they were sent home to die and now they were coming to me. I was their last hope. In the final decade of my clinic, many of my patients were told they would be dead months before I ever saw them. Often I referred to them (*behind their backs, of course*) as the "walking dead" just to keep myself and my staff smiling. At the very end of my clinic, the average patient was told they would be dead six months *before* I ever got to see them.

Anyway, on their first visit, I would take all of their tests results, pictures and very important papers and files, and throw it all in a big trash bin I had in my office. This was a very tense and intense moment. I had one woman hit me as hard as she could, knocking me right off of my examination stool! Usually, they would initially jolt towards the basket, often they would start to tremble, shake and start crying. Sometimes they would even wrestle me trying to get the papers back out of the bin, and if they did I would start ripping the papers up, and I always won. After all, they were sick, weak, and I am a 5th-degree black belt. And, I would eventually calm them down (sometimes it would take a half hour) and explain to them we were going to take a new approach to healing and getting well.

I would give them the next big scare by telling them that not only I had no idea what the heck was really wrong with them, nor could I understand most of their tests results, but worse, I had no idea how to heal their disease either!

Now they would always start crying, really crying, and usually sobbing with snot running out of their nose. After all, I was their last hope, their final shot, and even all of their relatives had warned them not to come see me and waste what little was left of their money. But, they came anyway and now they were falling into the abyss.

Again, I had just told them that I had no idea what was wrong with them, and also I had no idea how to heal their disease.

BUT, then I would tell them what I did know, which is how to create such an amazingly healthy lifestyle and amazingly healthy environment, that their body would HEAL ITSELF all on its own. And, it would do this better than any medical doctor or any top specialist could imagine.

BUT, the difference would be that we were never again going to talk about their disease, the name of it, or refer to any papers or test about their disease or go to any bullshit support groups. To support what? *Their having a disease?* NO. Instead we were going to focus on only one thing, the exact opposite, not *healing disease*, but GETTING HEALTHY! And, we were going to do this with such gusto, such aggressiveness, such intensity and so much positive energy, that their disease wouldn't stand a chance and it would LEAP out of their body. And, it did.

The Chinese have a saying, "Focus on the GOOD to Eliminate the BAD"—and, that is exactly what we did! And, did I see results, healings, miracles and smiles? Don't get me wrong, we did a lot of extremely hard work and paid a lot of dues to get these miracles, but we did it smiling and laughing all the way!

I will always remember one of my great teachers, Dr. John Christopher saying that if a patient vomited after drinking one of his herbal medicines, well, "They now have a cleaner stomach for the next dose". Intensify this 1,000 times, adding seizures, pain, blood, pus and rotting flesh, and my interns passing out (it *can get intense in the heat of healing*), but I never allowed one negative word to be uttered in my clinic, and forced my patients to learn 1,000 jokes, and become masters of positive thinking, positive affirmations and positive extremely healthy living. YES!

Step 3: Your First Detox
My 5-Day BOWEL Detox

So you can see, that I never focused on the disease itself.

Again, the sign in my office said:

"You can heal yourself of ANY disease or illness.

All you have to do is:

STOP doing what you did that made you sick, and

START doing what will create powerful health."

So, instead I first focused on getting my patients to STOP doing all of the things that caused their diseases in the first place. Then, where my programs came in, eating right, moving more, cleaning and stimulating the elimination organs, including Detoxification, this was starting new things, new programs, that would Create Powerful Health.

One of the first programs was Detoxification, and the first Detoxification Program was my Bowel Detox Program.

The main reason you must detoxify the body is simply because this retained toxic waste is a major factor in what is causing

your body to be physically stressed, immunologically stressed, blocked, and it is this toxic poison that is causing your body to breakdown, become irritated and inflamed, causing cellular degeneration and eventually to become ill and become diseased.

So, the first order of business is to cleanse and empty out any and all accumulated waste, toxins, poisons, chemicals, sludge, fat, grease, acids, mucous, bile, whatever—every bit of the waste in your body.

And, the best place to begin is the Bowel. Why? Simply because the way most of your body cleans and detoxifies itself, it does so by eventually dumping most of this toxic waste into your digestive and elimination tract, to be eliminated with your fecal matter. But a sluggish colon, that doesn't eliminate waste frequently and efficiently, doesn't send a message to your body to send more waste. A sluggish and dirty bowel causes your body to become a sluggish waste removal machine, because it knows if it detoxifies and purges out toxic material, it won't go anywhere—it cannot get out of you, and worse, *you may just re-absorb this toxic waste back into your body!*

So first stimulating, then cleansing, detoxifying, and then drawing out old waste from your bowel, empties, tones and strengthens your bowel—your major elimination organ—and then *encourages* your body to eliminate even more waste, even more deep rooted waste, from all of your other elimination channels.

Now, with any further Detoxification Programs that you do, any toxins that are dumped into your bowel will be eliminated rapidly and efficiently.

This is why Bowel Detoxification is the FIRST and most important step in any healing program and the FIRST Detoxification that EVERYONE needs to do.

What is so amazing, even to me after all of these years, is that when I would start ALL of my patients on STOPPING what was making them sick, and STARTING them on their healthy food and lifestyle programs, and do their very first of

my clinical Detox programs, their 5-Day Bowel Detox, THEY GOT WELL!

That's right! Over 80% of my patients, before I gave them any herbal medicine to address their specific complaints, HEALED THEMSELVES—their complaints were GONE—just by doing a thorough cleaning and detoxification of their bowel.

This shows the health-degenerating, negative power of your body being dirty and backed-up with accumulated fecal waste, toxins and poisons. It is such a powerful negative health-degenerating factor—this negative physical stress doesn't allow you to feel good and doesn't allow you to be well. And, it is this negative physiological stress of a dirty body that is causing it to break down, have little or no resistance to disease and then become diseased. So in a way, you could say that a clogged and dirty body is the root cause of all disease. In fact, I will say that!

BLOCKAGE: The Cause of All Dis-ease!

In my clinic I also had another sign: **"BLOCKAGE is the cause of all dis-ease!"** Think about it...

BLOCKAGE of blood is the cause of the #1 cause of death in America—heart attacks, strokes and circulatory disease. The blood vessels get blocked with fat, cholesterol, hard minerals and numerous other waste materials that are backed up in the body and eventually find their way to our coronary and cerebral arteries, block these arteries and kill us. This is what directly causes the #1 cause of death in America... BLOCKAGE!

BLOCKAGE of lymph and swollen and infected lymph nodes and nodules is found with Cancer, the #2 cause of all deaths in America. The lymph system is a system in your body that drains waste fluid from all organs and tissues and also allows your disease and infection fighting immune cells to travel where needed. When this system is blocked, waste builds up everywhere in your body and also blocks your immune system from healing you.

BLOCKAGE of your liver and gallbladder, caused by a high-fat animal-based diet, and an overexposure to toxic chemicals, causes your liver to fail and your gallbladder to get congested. Then, your liver stops doing its very important job of keeping your blood clean. This is also a contributing factor to the #2 cause of death in America... Cancer!

BLOCKAGE and breakdown of the nervous system is the cause behind all neurological diseases.

BLOCKAGE of blood and oxygen to the brain causes everything from Alzheimer's, dementia, depression, anxiety, memory loss, and even eyesight and hearing problems.

BLOCKAGE of waste removal by the elimination organs causes toxic waste to back-up in your body, and even in your BRAIN. I have literally seen this accumulation of yellow sludge in the brain, and read many pathology reports where the doctors referred to it as an after-effect of Alzheimer's disease and dementia. It's not an after-effect, it is the CAUSE of these diseases.

This brain sludge can also cause endless emotional disorders. I have witnessed many patients with moderate to severe and life crippling emotional disorders, from chronic clinical depression and dementia, to bipolar disorder and even schizophrenia, have amazing recoveries, simply by doing a Bowel Detox Program. It opens up their elimination channels, and therefore, removes toxic fecal waste from the bowel, the bloodstream and even the brain. After all, you cannot have sweet thoughts on a sour stomach!

Detoxification and Cleansing Programs could be called FLUSHING programs and the act of FLUSHING out your body **UNBLOCKS** your body by removing waste. And **UNBLOCKING** your body allows blood, lymph, immune cells, nerve electricity, nutrition, oxygen, even LOVE and everything else to flow back into the sick, irritated, inflamed, degenerated and diseased areas of your body and then… the healing begins.

"My Health Building Food Program is the best place for everyone to start. It is where I started, and where I started all of my patients."

CHAPTER 9

Dr. Schulze's 3 CLINICAL FOOD PROGRAMS

My Self-Discovery of Healthy Food

I started to modify what I ate when the doctors first told me I was dying. It was a year-long process of eliminating all foods that were contributing to my ill health and including new foods that would assist my body to repair and heal itself, and create powerful health.

At first I eliminated red meat, because a Zen Buddhist monk suggested it would be better for my heart. At 16, my cholesterol level was over 300, as I had been raised in a German family where we consumed blood for breakfast, lunch, dinner and even dessert. If it was bleeding, we ate it. And, if it was green, we didn't eat it, and neither did our family dog.

The monk suggested that red meat (beef) was full of fat that made my blood fatty, thicker, and therefore, harder for my weak, deformed heart to pump this blood around my body. This made complete sense. After all, it takes more pressure to pump the same amount of concrete than to pump water. So, I stopped eating all red meat and very soon I felt a lot better, lighter, and best yet, I had a lot less episodes of arrhythmia, palpitations and tachycardia with my heart.

Then, I learned that chicken had almost the exact same amount of cholesterol as beef. In fact, four ounces of white meat chicken (*even without the skin*) has as much cholesterol as four ounces of full-fat hamburger. So, chicken was gone now, too. Now, I was a fishy/vegetarian.

Soon fish was dumped to avoid the mercury, heavy metals, pollution and parasites, and now I was a full-fledged lacto, lacto, lacto, lacto, ovo, ovo, ovo, ovo vegetarian. I describe it this way simply because I lived almost exclusively on eggs and omelettes for breakfast, milkshakes and cheese sandwiches for lunch and the same for dinner. I was making my own yogurt and kefir and I had my own cultures, but still wasn't eating much fruit or vegetables.

Then, lo and behold, I realized that my cholesterol level was still sky-high just from the dairy products. So, I set out to discover what foods were high in cholesterol, and I discovered that ONLY animal foods contain cholesterol, and that there is NO cholesterol in any fruit, vegetable, nut, seed, grain or bean... NONE! So that was it. I was now going to cut out my eggs and all dairy products and throw my kefir culture in the compost. I was now a complete vegan!

The problem was... What the heck was I going to eat? When I cleaned my refrigerator out of all the milk, butter, cheese, yogurt, kefir, eggs, etc, there was nothing left in it but bread. I had some learning to do about being a vegan. It was hard at first, but I WANTED TO LIVE! So, a vegan food program it was, for me, and eventually for all of my patients, at least while they were healing their diseases.

Eliminating all animal food from my diet healed my heart, it literally saved my life, and also later in life, it saved the lives of my patients. **To this day, I use a vegan food program as the foundation to all three of my clinical healing food programs, to help people heal their diseases, regain their health and stay healthy.**

I am not going to get into the 100 reasons why a vegan food program is the best when you are healing yourself from any disease or creating powerful health, but I can assure you it is NOT a moral issue. I can't imagine the survival circumstance, but if I had to, to survive, I would kill a few people and eat them, and I would start with one of my ex-lawyers.

Seriously, my point is that I suggest a vegan/vegetarian food program as the foundation for all three of my food programs simply because it supplies you with the finest nutrition with none of the many negative side-effects of an animal-based diet. Again, it is NOT for moral reasons, it is strictly for health reasons. I could go into an eight-hour lecture right here about fat, cholesterol, infection, or steroid, growth hormone and antibiotic drug residues, or parasites and carcinogenic studies, but you have to simply take my word for it right here and now.

If you want more information, please read "Step #3: Vegan Food" from my book, *20 Powerful Steps to a Healhier Life*.

If you are trying to heal disease, any disease, and you are serious about it, or even trying to build the most powerful health, you do NOT want to be consuming any animals nor any animal by-products. I am not going to argue with you about your blood type, your ancestry or what tastes good to you. And, after you are healed, clean and feel great, if you want to go back and eat a burger and a milkshake, that is your business. **But, I would be bullshitting you plain and simple, if I told you that you could heal yourself from disease and build powerful health naturally—without doctors, drugs and hospitals—and still eat animals and animal products at the same time. You cannot! I have never seen this work and it didn't work in my clinic either. PERIOD!**

Now, since this is a book about detoxification, the same holds true here. If you are serious about detoxification and getting the most out of it, well, at least during your Detox routine, you need to refrain from ingesting anything that is toxic, does not contain fiber and is congesting and constipating. This just makes good common sense—why waste your time? We are trying to get the waste OUT, not plug you up. So, a Vegan/Vegetarian Food Program it is!

My 3 Food Programs Are:
#1 Juice Flushing
#2 Raw Food Program
#3 Health Building Food Program

They are all Vegan/Vegetarian.

The Juice Flushing Program is just pure water, herbal teas and fresh, organic, raw fruit and vegetable juice.

Benefits: It is the most powerful for cleansing, detoxifying, healing disease and creating powerful health. This is the best program to immediately go on if you are sick, ill or have any disease, and stay on it until you are well. It is also the food program that I generally suggest for everyone to do for the middle two to three days during any 5-Day Detox. And, if someone has a life-threatening illness or disease, this is the food program for them.

The Raw Food Program is any fruit or vegetable juice, just like the Juice Flushing Program, but you are also allowed to eat fresh fruits and vegetables and also sprouted grains, seeds, beans and raw nuts. Basically, anything that you can eat in its raw form is allowed.

Benefits: This is also a very powerful food program for cleansing, detoxifying, healing disease and creating powerful health. It is not as cleansing and detoxifying as the Juice Flushing Program, but at the same time it is more nourishing and health building than the Juice Flushing Program. This food program is good for detoxification and also good for healing disease and building health. It is a great transition food program between Juice Flushing and my Health Building Food Program. This is a great food program to begin and end a 5-Day Detox with, on days one and five, to transition from the Health Building Food Program to the Juice Flushing Program, and then back to the Health Building Food Program.

The Health Building Food Program is the general food program that I suggest people stay on for most of the year, in between flushing, Detox and Cleansing programs. It is my most adjustable and varied food program, where you can eat any foods, raw and cooked, in any shape or form, as long as they are vegan. This food program will build lasting health, strength and vitality.

Benefits: The benefits mirror the name—this food program BUILDS HEALTH! It floods your body with nutrition, it has the most varied choices of food, and the most substantial amounts of food.

My Health Building Food Program is the best place for everyone to start. It is where I started and where I started all of my patients. Unless a person is doing a Detox Program, or is sick or diseased, or is in immediate danger of dying, then this is the food program to be on.

Dr. Schulze's JUICE FLUSHING PROGRAM

Why Juice Flushing?

Juice Flushing gets MAXIMUM NUTRITION INTO your body and MAXIMUM WASTE OUT! It is the most powerful food program for Detoxification.

Whenever you don't feel well, whenever you feel sick, whenever you have pain, whenever you have a fever or inflammation, whenever you have any dis-ease or illness, **STOP EATING!!!**

When you are sick, the best way to assist your body to heal itself is to stop eating ALL solid food. Many foods can take eight hours or more to digest and this takes a lot of energy away from your body trying to heal itself—energy that can be better used in healing. It also takes a lot of blood to run your entire digestive system, blood that can be used more efficiently to heal you.

Also, Juice FLUSHING is the most powerful food program to open and stimulate your elimination organs and FLUSH the waste out of every cell in your body.

Juice Flushing is also a Natural Healing "Blood Transfusion". On many, many occasions, I would end up seeing one of my patients in the hospital, only to be told they were anemic. Whether it was from their cancer or a car crash where they had lost a lot of blood, I needed them to build more blood fast, and build powerful blood fast. The medical doctors were always amazed at how fast I could get their blood values and hemoglobin up with my fresh juice combinations. This is because fresh juice hardly has to be digested, and it is power-packed with live vitamins, minerals, amino acids, enzymes and the lifeblood of fruits and vegetables. Juice Flushing creates MIRACLES!

I had one woman who was so anemic from blood loss that they thought she might die. I brought the juicer right into her hospital room and made her my "Carrot, Beet and Beet Green Combo". In less than 12 hours, her hemoglobin count raised up to over that of a male count, and the doctors were shocked again. So Juice Flushing really gets **MAXIMUM NUTRITION IN.**

The reason I like to refer to this program as a FLUSH, instead of a FAST, is simply because the word "fast" seems like deprivation to me, where a FLUSH seems like you are drinking copious amounts of liquid, which is exactly what I want you to do. I wanted my patients and you, to get that the more you drink, the better.

Also, this program FLUSHES the poisons, toxins and waste right out of your body, out of every cell in your body. This food program gets **MAXIMUM WASTE OUT.**

Don't worry if you are getting enough calories, protein, calcium or anything. DON'T WORRY. I have personally done many 30-day juice flushes—and even 60-day juice flushes—and I have had terminally ill patients stay on juices for six months, even a year, and no one died. In fact, just the opposite, they THRIVED!

When you are Juice Flushing, **drink about one gallon of fresh juices and pure water every day.** If you get hungry, DRINK MORE. If you feel cold or weak, DRINK MORE. And, when you are in doubt, DRINK MORE!

What Foods Can You JUICE?

Just about anything. The first step is to get a great juicer. **It is an absolute MUST that you make ALL the juices yourself.** This is an important part of the process, so get a juicer.

Which Juicer

I have owned every type of juicer made, from centrifugal to extraction, to grating and hydraulic compression. They all work, but if I could have only one it would be the Champion, and my reason is simple. It ejects the pulp, so instead of spending a lot of your time opening up the juicer and cleaning all the pulp out, you can instead just keep juicing. So, you want a pulp-ejection juicer. Secondly, it's easy to clean, and my desire to be healthy is balanced by how long it takes to clean the damn juicer and a Champion has only a few parts and cleans easily. It is also strong, powerful and with minimal care it will still be juicing for your grandchildren years, even decades, from now. And, it is about $300.

There are many other types, again, stay away from the centrifugal because they have to be cleaned constantly. The ones that grate the fruit or veggies, and then squeeze the pulp in a hydraulic press are awesome (this is actually how I make my herbal extracts, but on a much bigger level), but these juicers can cost thousands of dollars, so usually I end up back with the Champion.

And, make sure that ALL of the produce that you juice is **Raw, Washed and Organically Grown.** If it isn't, then you are just putting more poisons right back into your body.

You can juice any fruit, and with the thicker foamier fruits like pineapple, you may want to add some water to thin it out. Don't forget to mix your fruits and make fruit juice blends. With vegetables, use your imagination, too. In spite of what some juice purists say, you can even mix some fruit and vegetable juices too, especially if this helps you to get them down. I have started a lot of kids, even adult kids, on "Carrot, Apple and Ginger". With kids, start with about 90% apple and 10% carrot, and then (as they begin to like it) slowly add more carrot. You will have everyone in the family drinking fresh juices, including carrot, and loving it in no time.

In the summer, I LOVE making watermelon juice. I juice the flesh, rind, seeds and all! It will make you pee your brains out; it is a powerful diuretic.

If you want to detoxify more, drink some wheatgrass juice or add a few ounces of it to 16-ounces of vegetable juice. And, if you have cancer, make your juice using cruciferous vegetables like broccoli, brussel sprouts, cauliflower, kale, etc. With these, a little goes a long way, so only add 1 or 2 ounces of them to start.

Make your juice your medicine. Speaking of medicine, add a little bit of fresh herbs as you are making your juice, like hot peppers, ginger, garlic, onions, horseradish and many of the aromatic greens. This is how I invented my SuperTonic. I wanted something I could make in the juicer.

For further information and a few juice recipes, see "Step 2: Fresh Juice" from my book, *20 Powerful Steps to a Healthier Life*.

Three Winning Tips About Juice Flushing

When Juice Flushing you can experience three things that are common, and so I wanted you to know about them before you experience them, so you know exactly how to handle them.

Feeling Cold: During Juice Flushing, you are taking in a lot less calories, so your body won't heat up as easily. It is natural to feel a little cooler once in a while, if not cold on occasion. Usually, this only lasts a few minutes. The cure for this is easy—it's called a sweater, sweatshirt or a jacket. When you are Juice Flushing, know that you can have an occasional period where you feel cold, so take along a warm piece of clothing, just in case this happens. Then, you will be fine, and again, this usually only lasts a short time.

Feeling Hungry: It is normal to have an occasional hunger "moment", if not a hunger "panic" or even see a mirage of a baked potato while you are driving down the highway. Seriously, you may have a moment where all of a sudden, out of nowhere, you are starving and want some solid food immediately. DO NOT EAT! The solution? Just drink more and keep drinking more liquid, until you are full. This will take care of the problem. It's not real. Remember, you can go months without any solid food, so just keep drinking and keep flushing.

Feeling Tired: Another normal feeling that can arise during a Juice Flush is all of a sudden, you feel very tired, if not exhausted. Again, this is one not to pay too much attention to. It is almost always gone in 5 or 10 minutes, and the next thing you know you have more energy, than you know what to do with. It is normal to have big energy spurts most of the time while juice flushing, and with an occasional moment of feeling tired once or twice a day. Don't fight it, take a break, even take a power nap, and the next thing you know, you will be energized again. I always remind people that after almost a month on juice flushing, I full contact kickboxed over 20 three-minute rounds and never got tired, and no one could touch me, and I was lightning fast and not tired at all.

Dr. Schulze's RAW FOOD PROGRAM

Why Raw Foods?

My Raw Food Program gets MORE NUTRITION INTO your body and MORE WASTE OUT! The Raw Food Program is more nutritious and more flushing that my **Health Building Food Program** that is next, but it is slightly less powerful at supplying nutrition and flushing you out than the previous **Juice Flushing Program.** It is my in-between food program.

My next food program, my Health Building Food Program, is the program that most of my patients, myself included, stayed on most of the year. But, occasionally when you want to get more nutrition into your body, clean up your body more, lose a few pounds and stimulate your elimination, then this **Raw Food Program** has more concentrated nutrition and will also stimulate more Detoxification. In my clinic, I referred to it as my ***Purifying*** Raw Foods Program, because that is exactly what it does, PURIFY your body.

I suggest that EVERYONE does this Raw Food Program for a minimum of one week every season, so a total of four weeks a year, MINIMUM!

It is especially great to follow this program when doing one of my seasonal **5-Day Detox Programs**. My patients that did a week of this **Raw Food Program** along with choosing one of my **5-Day Detox Programs** every season, four times a year, rarely got sick, if ever. That's PREVENTION!

Also, if you are going from my next food program, my Health Building Food Program, to do my Juice Flushing, unless you are having an emergency, it is better to stop at this food program for at least one day, and use this Raw Food Program, as a stepping stone, in between the Health Building Food Program and the Juice Flushing Program, to ease your way in and out of the Juice Flushing Program. So, at least do one day of this Raw Food Program when beginning and ending the Juice Flushing Program.

What Foods Can You EAT?

This program consists of eating only foods that you can eat RAW. Basically, any food that has not been heated, like fresh fruit and fruit juices, vegetables and vegetable juices, raw nuts and seeds, and sprouted beans, seeds and grains. I like to start my morning with fresh fruit, as it is the easiest and quickest to digest. So, in the morning, you can consume water, herbal teas, fruit juices and raw fruit. If you have blood-sugar problems or if many juices seem too sweet to you, then you can simply dilute them 50/50 with clean, pure water. You can also make SMOOTHIES in your blender or Vita-Mix.

As the midday comes around, switch to vegetables and consume vegetable juices and raw vegetables. You can also dilute your vegetable juices 50/50 with pure water. Then, towards the evening (after 6 pm) go back to fruit juices and fresh fruit. Remember, ALL of your juices, fruit and vegetables should be fresh, organic and RAW. Again, it doesn't make any sense to consume foods that are grown with poisons and sprayed with poisons, when you are trying to get the poisons OUT of your body.

Look, I am not going to list 100 fruits and 100 vegetables here. Make this fun, make great fruit smoothies, make great veggie salads, **make raw dressings with raw vinegar, fresh citrus juice, avocado, onions, garlic, tomatoes, raw nuts like sunflower seeds and almonds** and try all of the different sprouts. A big key is to HAVE FUN! Don't torture yourself. Make this a fun, raw food adventure! Find and eat fruit, vegetables, nuts and sprouts that you have never had, or haven't had in years.

If it helps, there are hundreds of Raw Food UN-COOK books out there in health food stores and most major bookstores.

I even take various vegetables, some herbs and water and liquify them in my Vita-Mix to make raw soups... YUM!

Just EAT IT RAW!

For further information see "Step 4: Live Food" from my book, *20 Powerful Steps to a Healthier Life*.

Dr. Schulze's HEALTH BUILDING FOOD PROGRAM

Why the Health Building Food Program?

This food program is the best day-to-day food program to do most of the year. It is nutritious and will not overwhelm or overload your body with toxins, nor is it congesting, constipating and it won't lead to blockage. It will generally build vitality, strength and health.

As I mentioned previously, all three food programs that I use are vegan.

I don't mean to insult your intelligence or be redundant, but you would be as surprised as I was to see how many people thought that I certainly didn't mean lobster, or "Aren't oysters supposed to be healthy?" or "Surely you didn't mean goat's milk, yogurt or kefir? Aren't they health foods?" I even had one patient from Kazakhstan in the southern part of the old USSR who was drinking curdled horse milk for the first month and a half on his program until I discovered it. He said, "Well, it wasn't on your list of don'ts," *and he was right*. So after that experience, I actually had an entire 8.5" x 11" sheet of paper for each patient, which listed by name every type of animal food that existed and all animal by-products known, from sheep's brains and steak tartare to haggis and braun for the Scotsmen. I would still add a new animal food every month or so when I discovered a new one. So, the bottom line is that I cannot be clear enough on this issue.

What I mean is that all three of my food programs, including this **Health Building Food Program**, are totally vegan/vegetarian, with no meat, fish, fowl, eggs or dairy products. To be very specific, I mean no cows, pigs, boars, lamb, goats, horses, deer, elks, bears, turkeys, chickens, ducks, game birds, ostrich, fish, clams, mussels, lobsters, abalones, oysters, shrimps, scallops, calamari, conch, sushi, reptiles, chicken eggs, any eggs, cow's milk, goat's milk, any animal parts, muscles, organs, skin, blood or animal milks or animal fluids of any kind!

Again, as I said at the beginning, this is NOT some moral or "save the whales" issue here. It is purely that when I design the best food program for my patients, based on the fact that the majority of them were dying from heart and circulatory disease, followed closely by cancer, well, the mountains of evidence that has been piling up over the past two or three decades linking animal food to both of these diseases, from cow's milk and breast cancer, to red meat and prostate cancer, to charred beef and colon cancer, to ALL cholesterol from animal foods blocking arteries to the heart and brain, well, I cannot condone the consumption of any animal foods on any health program.

Now having said that, no one ever dropped dead immediately from eating one hamburger. But, my point is simply that animal food is NOT health or healing food. And, that the American animal-based diet is way out of control and way out of balance, to the point where the over-consumption of animal foods can be linked to being at least a contributing cause, if not *the* cause, of almost every major disease.

The Chinese eat both beef and pork and still maintain an average cholesterol level of 122 with little incidence of coronary artery disease. But, they only consume a pound of meat a week per family of four. *That is only about 1/2 ounce of animal per person per day or 1/5 ounce per meal.* That is why it is hard to find the meat in most Chinese food, because it is in such a small portion compared to the rice and vegetables. As the Chinese society modernizes, along with Americanizing their diet, I am sure we will see the animal consumption increase along with the incidence of heart disease and cancer.

I can make this statement with much authority from my clinical experience. In my clinic, I had many patients who were immigrants, whose parents still lived in the "old country". What I found interesting, is that many of my immigrant patients had diseases in their fifties, that were unheard of in the village where they were born. And more often than not, their parents were still alive and healthier in their eighties and nineties, and were still living in the "old country" and didn't have any of these same diseases. They were healthier than their children who were now living in America. These "new country" diseases could be simply attributed to living the American Dream, and eating in the American Way.

I know that up to now I have talked a lot about the disease and death caused by eating animals. But eating a food program of fruit, vegetables, grains, beans, legumes, seeds, nuts and sprouts has an equal and opposite *upside*. A healthy food program is the foundation of Natural Healing. Notice that I didn't say ***a*** foundation, I said **THE** foundation.

Eating this type of food gives you maximum nutrition with the minimum digestive effort, without any toxic pollution of your body. There are also many other attributes to this vegetarian food program, like fiber. Fiber has many healing benefits, including helping your entire digestive tract work better, especially your bowel elimination. Absolutely NO animal food contains ANY fiber. It only exists in the plant world. Interestingly, NO plant food contains any cholesterol. None. ZERO. So, the Health Building Food Program, as with all of my food programs, is HIGH fiber and ZERO cholesterol.

My **Health Building Food Program** is also my most lenient and varied food program. That is why it is the best one on which to start. It is also the best maintenance food program, the one you will usually stay on about 48 weeks a year. My patients who followed this type of food program maintained powerful health.

The only exception would be that if you became ill, you would immediately stop the **Health Building Food Program** and begin the **Raw Food Program**. If you were really ill, you would stop all solid food and move immediately onto my **Juice Flushing Program.**

Again, the Health Building Food Program is designed to supply your body with optimum nutrition in a manner that is easy to digest and assimilate. The food on this program is not toxic or congestive to your body in any way, but will not generally initiate a cleanse or detoxification either.

What Foods Can I Eat?

The Health Building Food Program consists of all fruits, vegetables, grains, beans, legumes, seeds, nuts and sprouts. They can be raw, sprouted, steamed or cooked. At first, to the novice, this may not seem like a lot of food or food choices, but you will see that there is an almost unlimited array of food choices and menu options on this program. Veggie chili, soy cheese veggie burgers, spaghetti and baked potatoes are totally legal on this program. As you begin to use your imagination, you will find that this food program is totally sustainable and easily followed. Saying that, I would always steer my patients into choosing simple healthy foods and leave the health food *merchandise* for the weekends and parties.

As you are working toward making this food program your new way of life, it is important to be very receptive and positive about the new types of food that you may eat and be imaginative and inventive about the preparation of them. Most people don't eat a raw, cold hamburger on a plate with nothing else on it—so don't do this with a veggie burger either! Remember to enjoy herbs and spices and all the many great sauces and condiments that are available in the health food store and also make your own. Additionally, remember to use your imagination, and most importantly, keep your sense of humor.

Visit the health food store more, like a museum, and always leave yourself plenty of time to browse around. There are new products coming out every week and many of them are great. Some are not so great and some you might be better off steaming and eating the box and throwing out the contents, but in any case, try everything!

I used to take my patients on a "field trip", in one of their first five or ten visits, and meet them at the local health food store and take them shopping. I would talk to them in every isle explaining some of the foods and how I like to prepare them. My patients at first thought this was silly and a waste of time and money, but soon discovered that this was one of their favorite doctor visits.

Enjoy yourself and make this a positive, exciting adventure into your new, healthy way of living. Everything sold in a health food store is not necessarily healthy, but it will almost always be better than its counterpart in a regular grocery store (less fat, salt, sugar, artificial colorings, flavorings and dangerous preservatives, etc). Keep reading the product labels, even in the health food store.

Note: Remember, it's not what you do on holidays, New Year's Eve, your birthday or Saturday night that counts. It's what you do six days a week that determines your level of health.

The Health Building Morning

I always suggest starting each day with 8 ounces of pure water. This will flush your digestive tract of any leftover digestive juices and food. It is also the best way to lubricate and cleanse your body. A great time to do it is when you are **break**ing the **fast: break-fast.**

Next, I suggest some type of blender drink. To gulp down a piece of toast or eat some cereal first thing in the morning sets our digestive tract off to six hours of hard labor. This is why most people feel tired all morning and then need coffee to keep them going. Start your day off instead with a nutritional morning drink that assimilates fast, getting your blood packed with vitamins, minerals, enzymes, amino acids and hundreds of other nutritional substances that give you energy.

For over 40 years now, I have been playing around, making hundreds of different variations of my morning blender drink. Most people are not as obsessed as I am with nutrition. I add a little bit of this and that and make some powerful morning nutritional blender drinks.

But in the clinic, making morning drinks for my patients was a very serious business. Many of my patients were anemic from leukemia and other diseases. If they didn't get their nutrition, they could be dead by nightfall. I had a couple problems I had to overcome with these patients.

First, they were so sick that they had very little, if any, digestive ability. Their digestive ability was poor because of liver cancer, pancreatic cancer, chronic stomach ulcers, bowel disease and many had literally burned out their digestive tracts from years on extremely harsh medical drugs.

Secondly, even if they could digest a vitamin pill, they didn't stand a chance at assimilating it. After all, it's not really how much you take of a particular nutrient that makes the difference. The question is how much of that nutrient you ***assimilate*** and get into your bloodstream and to the dying cells that need it.

So to keep these patients alive, many years ago in my clinic, I did lots of experimentation with juicing, juicers, juices and juice combinations.

Without a doubt, fresh, organic juice kept my patients alive. I have said it many times—it is like a **Natural Healing blood transfusion.**

Regardless, some of my patients still needed something even more nutritionally concentrated, potent and powerful than just juice. That is when I started investigating food supplements that were extremely high in particular vitamins and minerals. I was also looking at single-cell micro herbs like spirulina, blue-green algae, chlorella and non-fermentable saccharomyces cervisiae nutritional yeast. I searched out super foods that are the highest in particular nutrients, but that are also *single-celled*, ones that can be assimilated into your blood from your mouth, before they even reach your intestines. I knew immediately that these foods and herbs were the missing answer that I needed for my sickest patients.

I would add beets and spinach for iron to get their anemic blood fortified and get their hemoglobin count up. I would add dulse and seaweeds to get them their minerals, and trace minerals, and add wheatgrass to clean their blood, and alfalfa and barley grass to fortify their blood. I added citrus peels, so they not only got Vitamin C, but also the Vitamin C-complex nutrients like rutin, hesperidin and bioflavonoids, and numerous other herbs to blast their body with nutrition. It saved lives.

So, I cannot over emphasize the importance of starting out your Health Building day with a great, imaginative, tasty, power-packed, nutritional morning blender drink.

For further information, see "Step 3: Vegan Food" from my book, *20 Powerful Steps to a Healthier Life*.

"The United States Department of Agriculture states that the average American vegetarian consumes 150% of their needed protein requirements."

BONUS CHAPTER

QUESTIONS AND FEARS ABOUT BECOMING A VEGETARIAN

Most of my patients were in the entertainment industry, whether in front of the camera, behind it or on stage. They worked long hours and put out a lot of energy. Many of my patients were professional athletes, dancers, body builders, yoga teachers and people with very active lifestyles. Almost daily, I was asked the same questions regarding being a vegetarian:

Is there enough PROTEIN in a vegetarian diet?

Will I have enough ENERGY?

Where will I get my CALCIUM without drinking milk or using dairy products?

I would like to address these three questions...

PROTEIN:

In regard to necessary protein consumption, a vegetarian diet has an overabundance. This brings up three very interesting protein facts:

#1: Any food program or diet that has sufficient caloric intake to sustain human life has also been proven to have sufficient amounts of protein. In fact, it is impossible to create a food program that has enough calories, but that is deficient in protein.

#2: High protein was a misguided nutritional fad of the 1950s. Many erroneously believed that a healthy person should consume 75 to 100 grams of protein a day. Today, it is understood that all of this protein actually created many diseases and made many people sick. A low-protein diet is now known to be the safest, healthiest and the most effective for longevity.

Interestingly, most of this supposedly scientific (and very wrong) high-protein dietary advice has now been traced back to the overzealous promoters at the beef and dairy industries. A similar example is that, in the 1930s, cigarettes were proclaimed by medical doctors to soothe throat inflammation—an advertisement promoted by the cigarette manufacturers. And, white-refined sugar was proclaimed an official food group (again, by medical doctors) promoted by the sugar industry. The Beef Advisory Board and the American Dairy Council have supplied most of the nutritional information we have relied on for the past 100 years, so we have not been getting facts, we have been getting advertising. Consequently, most of what we think we know about nutrition, and even what doctors say about nutrition, is actually nutritional lies developed by marketing executives.

#3: In a book by Frances Moore Lappe, the protein issue was again misguided. In this book, the author stated that you must eat complete proteins and, if you don't, then you must combine proteins in the same meal (like beans and rice) that add up to all of the eight essential amino acids making up a complete protein. This is simply hogwash. It has been scientifically disproved and additionally, even the author has now retracted this bad theory, but I still hear people every day spouting this nonsense. It goes to prove one thing, the old proverb, that "an old *lie*, is stronger than a new *truth*".

In the last 20 years, teams of medical researchers from Harvard, The American Dietetic Association, The American Medical Association and most other major conservative medical groups have studied the vegetarian diet. All of them came to the same conclusion. The vegetarian diet was "well above sufficient" in

protein and all other essential nutrients, even for pregnant women, growing children and teenagers.

So I hope we can put this protein issue to rest, forever!

ENERGY:

As far as the energy vs. protein intake issue, it seems to be a psychological issue, not a physiological one. In other words, it seems to be all in people's minds.

It appears that all the brainwashing by the Beef Advisory Board and the American Dairy Council has paid off again, as with the protein issue. **Many people seem to feel that protein gives us quick energy, but there is no scientific data or evidence to substantiate this feeling**. Protein (animal or vegetable) is essential for growth, repair and building new tissue, but it is complex carbohydrates, starch and sugars that give us energy. This is why many professional athletes, especially marathon runners, practice carbohydrate loading. They tend to maintain a very high carbohydrate diet in the days before an athletic competition or extensive workout. It is mainly complex carbohydrates, especially grains and vegetables, which your body converts to glycogen and stores for future energy needs. When needed, your body converts this glycogen to the sugar glucose, which is needed for muscular work, muscular contraction and energy.

In my clinic, I heard many people say that they used to be vegetarians, but they had to go back to eating meat again because they needed more *protein or more energy*. There is absolutely no scientific or medical basis for this phenomenon and after ~~interrogating~~, I mean interviewing, these patients, I always discovered that it was simply because the patient just wanted to eat meat again.

It may have been a comfort food for them or just a family tradition, but in this day and age, it is not cool anymore to say, "I started eating veal again, because my family is Italian and it makes me feel warm and fuzzy all over." It is much more politically correct (but scientifically *incorrect*) to just say, "I didn't have enough energy" or "I needed more protein". Or the newest bull: "I'm an O-blood type and I am supposed to eat meat."

CALCIUM:

And finally, the calcium issue. Calcium is needed by the body to build strong bones and teeth and to assist in numerous other extremely important metabolic functions. Our bones are comprised of about 85% calcium. Bone deterioration and brittleness seems to be caused by two major factors. First, not enough easy-to-assimilate calcium in our diets (like vegetables instead of dairy products, oyster shell calcium and ground-up rock calcium) and, here we go again, too much protein intake.

I am not going to write an in-depth metabolic essay here on how protein *intake* negatively affects your calcium *uptake*, but let me just tell you the basics.

When you consume a food that contains calcium, your body digests it and the calcium enters into your blood. After an amount of time, if there is excess calcium in your blood that you don't need, it is taken out of your blood and deposited into your bones. Your bones and skeletal system not only structurally support your body, but they also serve as a calcium depository and calcium storage reserve.

The metabolic downside of consuming too much protein is that in order to metabolize this protein, your kidneys remove your blood calcium and you urinate it away and it doesn't get a chance to be deposited into your bones. This is simply why meat eaters have double the bone loss and osteoporosis than vegetarians.

While misinformed doctors and animal industry advertisements tell women to ingest MORE calcium and animal food like dairy products to treat and prevent osteoporosis, the real metabolic solution is to simply consume LESS protein. This is why milk is NOT a good choice as a calcium supplement. Because it is also